Intermittent Fasting

The Ultimate Guide To Enhance Brain Health, Lose
Unwanted Fat, And Prolong Lifespan

*(Maintaining A Normal Blood Glucose Level And Efficient
Weight Management)*

Winston-Francois Fleury

TABLE OF CONTENT

Introduction

In addition to weight loss, intermittent fasting has been shown to have a variety of other long-lasting benefits. When it comes to our diet, we frequently overlook the most crucial aspect. We frequently ask ourselves, "What should I eat?" It appears that we frequently, if not constantly, ask ourselves this question, but "When should I eat?" is a far more significant inquiry. We have neglected to pose this question to ourselves.

When we eat, our body produces the hormone insulin. Insulin regulates how our bodies metabolise food. Part of the food we eat is utilised for energy, while the rest is stored as fat, which contains potential energy.

Numerous meals cause an increase in insulin production, and when insulin levels are maintained for an extended period of time, insulin resistance develops.

At this point, weight gain and ultimately obesity begin to emerge.
Maintaining low insulin levels over an extended period of time is therefore required to prevent insulin resistance; however, how can this be accomplished?

Currently, the solution should be readily apparent. To stop this, a period of total fasting is required.

Considering that every meal raises insulin levels, it follows that no food could naturally lower them. I am discussing intermittent fasting. You do not need to ask yourself, "Am I going to starve to death? " because this is not a famine.

Chapter 1: The Mechanisms Of
Intermittent Fasting

Although insulin is technically a storage hormone, it serves a regulatory purpose. Increased insulin levels prevent weight loss because they cause the body to burn food for energy rather than stored fat.

After three to five hours, the digestive process is complete, and the body enters the post-absorptive state. The post-absorptive state can last anywhere between eight and twelve hours. After this duration, your body enters a state of fasting. Your insulin levels are low because your body has completed digesting your meal, making stored fat readily available for oxidation.

Intermittent fasting allows the body to enter an advanced fat-burning state when compared to the standard "three meals a day" diet. While fasting, since there is no food left for the body to use as fuel, stored fat is burned instead. This factor alone explains why many people experience quick results with intermittent fasting without changing their exercise routines, the amount or type of food they consume, or their eating habits.

Simply put, they are altering the timing and frequency of their meals. Getting used to an intermittent fasting programme may take some time once you've begun. Don't lose hope! Immediately resume your intermittent fasting schedule if you make a mistake. Stay away from self-criticism and guilt-tripping. Negative self-talk delays your return to your routine.

No one expects you to change your lifestyle perfectly on your first attempt; it requires effort. If you are not accustomed to going long periods without food, intermittent fasting will take some getting used to. You will quickly master it if you select the optimal strategy, maintain concentration, and keep a positive outlook.

The intermittent fast is an effective diet strategy, unlike some of the other diets you may try. It aids weight loss by taking advantage of how the body functions. When hearing about fasting, it is natural to feel apprehensive. You may believe it will be too challenging because you will go days or weeks without eating (and who has the willpower to do that, even if they want to lose weight).

Not only are one-week fasts extremely difficult, but they are also harmful to the body. If you fast for too long, your body will enter starvation mode frequently. Assuming you are in a period of limited food supply, your body will attempt to conserve calories and assist you in retaining as much fat and calories as possible. It implies that, in addition to being hungry, you are also preventing yourself from losing weight.

Because you will not be fasting for so long that your body enters starvation mode, you should be fine with how this intermittent fast functions in starvation mode. It ceases weight loss, and intermittent fasting is effective. Instead, it extends the fast just long enough to boost your metabolism.

The intermittent fast prevents the body from entering starvation mode after a few hours without food (usually no more than 24ish hours). Instead, it will utilise the available calories. If you consume the appropriate number of calories for the day, your body will switch to using its fat reserves. By adhering to an intermittent fasting routine, you force your body to burn fat at a faster rate without exerting more effort.

CHAPTER FOUR

What Is the Five-Two Diet Plan? How It Can Support Weight Loss And Its Health Benefits

This method is significantly more effective than counting calories.

Intermittent fasting has become a popular strategy for dietary improvement and weight loss. In case you were wondering, periodic fasting is followed by a return to a normal eating schedule. With so many options available, such as the 16:8 diet, it is simple to find one that works for you. You may have heard of the 5:2 diet if you're searching for an alternative approach. It allows you to consume whatever you want five days per week, but requires calorie restriction on the other two.

Two days per week, you consume approximately 25 percent fewer calories than usual."

Between 1,600 and 2,400 calories per day should be consumed by women. However, a physically active woman will require more. Consequently, you would consume 400–600 calories on fasting days.

The remaining five days of the week consist of business as usual. On the 5:2 diet, participants halve their weekly caloric intake in order to lose weight.

As long as you adhere to the calorie limits, you can eat whatever you want; however, the 5:2 Diet recommends consuming a lot of vegetables and small portions of lean meat, fish, and eggs. Additionally to broths! Low-calorie, satiating soups are a boon for dieters.

Chapter 2: How Well Does The 5:2 Diet Work For Losing Weight?

A calorie deficit of 3,500 per week is typically used to achieve a healthy weight loss rate of one to two pounds per week. After 12 months on the 5:2 diet, participants lost roughly the same amount of weight as those who followed a more conventional diet plan. In contrast, 5:2 dieters reported better outcomes than their normal diet counterparts.

In most cases, you will begin to see results within the first three weeks of the 5:2 diet.

It is up to you to determine whether this method of weight loss is sustainable.

Is It Healthy To Use The 5:2 Diet?

I believe that it does. The 5:2 diet is safe for adults to try because 500 calories is relatively low and nearly equivalent to one meal per day. Due to the fact that children's bodies are still growing and require more calories, it is unhealthy for them and unsafe for pregnant women.

The 5:2 diet should not be followed by individuals with a history of binge eating or dietary restriction. If you suffer from migraines and have discovered that skipping meals can worsen the pain, or if you are an intense gym-goer who sometimes forgets to eat before a workout, the same rule applies.

Additionally, while fasting on consecutive days is acceptable, you should not go without food for more than two days.

Chapter 3: How Dissimilar Is The Fast Diet From The 5:2 Diet, And What Similarities Exist?

There are striking differences between these two diets.

Regarding the Fast 800, for instance, you will have less flexibility.

To lose weight while following "The Fast 800" diet, one must consume no more than 800 calories per day for at least two weeks.

If you are close to your ideal weight, adopt the Mediterranean diet and restrict your caloric intake to 800 calories on two days per week.

One of the ways in which the Fast 800 is more difficult is because of the stricter early limits.

The 5:2 diet is, in my opinion, more sustainable in the long run than the Fast 800 diet.

If weight loss is your objective, you may wish to consider the 5:2 diet.

However, it is prudent to consult your physician first to rule out any underlying health conditions.

If you are underweight or have a history of eating disorders, it is not a good idea to fast unless you have spoken with a trained medical professional beforehand.

Ought Women to Fast?

There is evidence to suggest that women may not experience the same health benefits from intermittent fasting as men.

For example, research conducted in 2005 revealed that it increased insulin sensitivity in males while decreasing blood sugar management in females.

In rats, intermittent fasting can cause female rats to become masculinized, malnourished, and infertile, as well as miss their periods.

There are multiple anecdotal accounts of women whose menstrual periods ceased when they began intermittent fasting (IF) and resumed normalcy when they resumed their previous eating habits.

Due to the aforementioned factors, caution should be exercised by women who engage in intermittent fasting.

They must adhere to various recommendations, such as initiating the practise gradually and discontinuing it immediately if complications, such as amenorrhea, arise (absence of menstruation).

Consider postponing your attempt at intermittent fasting if you struggle with fertility, are attempting to conceive, or if both of these apply to you. This pattern of eating is probably not the best option for women who are pregnant or nursing.

Chapter 4: Some Methods For Intermittent Fasting That Are Backed By Research

There is no universal strategy for intermittent fasting, as it can be practised in a number of different ways. Individuals should experiment with different styles to determine which best suits their preferences and lifestyle.

Regardless of the type of intermittent fasting, prolonged fasting can be challenging if the body is unprepared. It is possible that these weight loss methods will not work for everyone.

With the likelihood that a person is prone to disordered eating, these techniques may exacerbate their undesirable relationship with food.

Before attempting any form of fasting, people with health conditions such as diabetes should consult a physician.

On days when you are not fasting, you must consume a balanced and nutritious diet.

Professional assistance is available to customise a plan for intermittent fasting and avoid potential pitfalls, if necessary. Continue reading to learn about seven distinct intermittent fasting methods.

Chapter 1: What, Precisely, Is A Hormone?

Chemical messengers, hormones influence mental, physical, and emotional health. It is essential for controlling appetite, weight, and mood, among other things. Changes in hormones and growth factors associated with increased food intake and obesity influence the regulation of genes involved in cellular processes such as proliferation, differentiation, and DNA repair, resulting in cell growth despite the accumulation of mutations. Cancer, survival, and multiplication Indeed, in numerous model organisms, the growth hormone/insulin growth factor-1 (GH/IGF-1)/insulin pathway and its downstream effectors promote ageing and/or age-associated diseases, such as cancer. It has been demonstrated that nutritional restriction has a substantial effect on hormone and growth factor levels, delaying the onset of age-related diseases and extending lifespan. This article summarises the effects of various nutritional intervention strategies on cell damage, ageing, and cancer.

Normally, your body produces adequate amounts of each hormone required for various processes to maintain health. On the other hand, a sedentary lifestyle and a Western diet can affect the hormonal environment. In addition, specific hormone levels decline with age, with some individuals experiencing a greater decline than others. You will lose weight, but a nutritious diet and other healthy lifestyle habits can help you feel and perform better by improving your hormonal health.

Hormones are complex, but there are four hormones that, especially in women, make weight loss extremely challenging. Here is a list of hormones, their effects on weight and fat burning, and at least one simple way to rebalance each hormone.

1. Estrogen Unbalance

Estrogen is a female hormone that nourishes and lubricates the breasts and hips of women. Men are also affected, albeit to a much lesser extent. However, both men and women are susceptible to oestrogen overload. This indicates that you have an excess of oestrogen in your body, despite being in menopause. Following menopause, the ovaries and adrenal glands continue to produce oestrogen (Estrogen levels fall after menopause, but oestrogen dominance can be maintained even if progesterone levels are extremely low.) Estrogen, along with other hormones, influences our responses to food, beverages, and supplements. Simply put, oestrogen dominance is the primary reason why women struggle to lose weight more than men, regardless of age.

How to manage- Consume one pound of vegetables to lower oestrogen levels (which helps her lose weight). Vegetable fibre aids in the elimination of oestrogen and does not circulate in the body like bad karma. Women should consume 35-45 grammes of fibre per day, while men should consume 40-50 grammes per day. To reach your goal without feeling bloated, gradually increase your fibre intake by 5 grammes per day. Additionally, eating more plants displaces meat consumption. This is vital for two important reasons. First, meat contributes significantly to climate change. Second, rapid changes in industrial agriculture and cultural expectations have outpaced our genetic adaptability over the past century.

Simply put, our DNA-based biology is incompatible with contemporary meat. Women are particularly susceptible to the estrogenic effects of meat. There is a complex connection between meat and oestrogen. Red meat raised conventionally increases the likelihood of excess oestrogen. There are compelling reasons to limit your consumption of conventional meat, but I'm not suggesting you must give up meat forever. It was effective, and we observed significantly superior results in men. Even when grass-fed, there have been no randomised trials in favour of or against eating meat. There is none.

There are compelling reasons to limit your consumption of conventional meat, though I am not advocating a total abstinence from meat consumption. Paleo is effective for some but not all women, and I have observed significantly better results in men. There are no randomised controlled trials supporting or opposing meat consumption, including pastured meat. Unfortunately, no high-quality evidence suggests that eating meat is healthier than eating plant-based protein, seafood, or poultry.

Insulin overdose

An estimated one in two Americans has diabetes, which is a combination of diabetes and obesity. If you are obese or underweight (normal weight with too little fat mass), your insulin will become out of control and your cells will die as they become hormonally insensitive. Fat accumulates as a result of its breakdown. Insulin has no effect. Your hormones and weight loss are out of your control.

Cortisol is produced in response to stress, and the majority of us are constantly stressed. When discussing hormonal imbalance and weight gain, all roads lead back to cortisol. The majority of us recognise that excessive cortisol is detrimental to our appearance and sanity, but common sense does not always translate into practise. Over time, fat accumulates and causes havoc. It primarily accumulates as visceral fat, the most dangerous type of fat, in the abdomen. High cortisol levels are also associated with binge eating and sugar cravings, which can lead to overeating of unhealthy foods like cookies and processed foods.

How to Recover - To restore cortisol, you must abstain from caffeine. Avoid caffeine for the next week to improve your sleep and stress levels. Prioritively, from coffee to half-café. Then, combine equal parts coffee and green tea. If desired, then switch from green to white tea. Replace your coffee with a steaming mug of lemon- and cayenne-seasoned hot water.

Adiponectin deficiency

Adiponectin is a hormone that assists in fat metabolism. It is contained by adipocytes and encased by the ADIPOQ gene. It regulates glucose levels and the breakdown of fatty acids. Some individuals are genetically predisposed to produce insufficient amounts of this hormone, and when levels drop, body fat percentage increases. The brain is crucial when it comes to weight loss resistance, and there is a secret connection between adipose tissue and the central nervous system, both of which contribute to weight gain.

Chapter 1: When and How

If you are performing intermittent fasting, you must adhere to your daily fasting and eating windows. Less emphasis is placed on WHAT to eat, though it remains crucial.

In essence, the best foods to consume during intermittent fasting are the best foods to consume in general. Included among them are avocado, potatoes, cruciferous vegetables, fish, seafood, whole grains, nuts, and fermented foods. Additionally, remembering to drink water daily is essential.

While attempting to lose weight, you should prioritise nutrient-dense foods such as fruits, vegetables, whole grains, nuts, beans, seeds, dairy, and lean proteins.

Almost every vital organ in your body requires water for optimal health. It would be foolish to exclude this item from your fast. Your organs play an important role in maintaining your life.

Each individual must consume a different amount of water based on their gender, height, weight, level of physical activity, and environment. The colour of your urine, however, is a reliable indicator. It must always be a pale yellow hue.

Dehydration can cause headaches, fatigue, and dizziness, and dark yellow urine is indicative of this condition.

Only water, coffee, and other calorie-free beverages are permitted during the fast. When unsure whether a particular food will break your fast, it is best to confirm its nutritional information online.

When you eat is primarily determined by the fasting time you've selected; ensure that your fasting times coincide with a schedule that works for you, and start slowly until you're completely acclimated to the lifestyle.

It is not advisable to do too much; instead, focus on a single activity so that you can improve. Combining intermittent fasting with other weight loss or extreme methods is not recommended. The foundation of weight loss is a calorie deficit. Intermittent fasting offers a simpler approach with a wealth of additional health benefits.

Doing too much at once will cause you to become overwhelmed and stressed, which may cause you to gain weight rather than lose it.

When breaking your fast, ensure that you begin with soups and drinks that are easy on the digestive system so as not to overwork it after a long period without food.

This will help you avoid the bloating and stomach aches that some people experience when they eat their heavier meals and foods first.

Chapter 6: What Is A Fast? And What Is The Advantage For You?

Fasting is not a novel idea. Fasting has been practised by humans for centuries. But what is fasting, and why has it recently gained such popularity? The act of abstaining from food and drink for a period of time is known as fasting. There are numerous reasons why people fast, but the most common is weight loss.

In recent years, fasting has gained popularity due to numerous studies demonstrating its ability to aid in rapid weight loss, burn fat, and improve health. In one study, participants who fasted lost significantly more weight than those who did not fast.

Prior to beginning a fast, it is essential to know how to do it properly and safely.

It is essential to understand that fasting is distinct from starvation. Starvation occurs when a person lacks access to food or chooses to abstain from eating, whereas fasting is a deliberate decision to abstain from eating for a predetermined period of time. It is also essential to ensure that you consume enough nutrients and calories during mealtimes.

There is no standard duration or frequency for fasting. Some individuals fast for an entire day at a time, while others may fast for multiple days in a week or even alternate days.

Voluntary abstinence from food and drink for a predetermined time period constitutes fasting. Particularly, intermittent fasting is characterised by alternating periods of fasting and eating. Fasting has been practised for centuries for religious, spiritual, and health-related reasons. Ancient Greek physicians prescribed fasting for a variety of illnesses, and Hippocrates believed that "to eat when ill is to feed your illness." In religions such as Christianity, Islam, Hinduism, and Buddhism, religious leaders have also fasted to seek a closer relationship with their deities.

In more recent times, fasting has been utilised as a method of weight loss. In his book The Fasting Cure, published in the early 1900s, physician and nutritionist Lorenzo Costa advocated intermittent fasting for weight loss. In his book Fasting for Health and Long Life, journalist and health writer Herbert M. Shelton popularised water fasting as a means of weight loss and disease treatment.

During World War II, when food was scarce or rationed, fasting was also utilised. This led to the creation of popular weight-loss diets such as the grapefruit diet and cabbage soup diet, in which individuals restricted their food intake to specific foods or food groups.
This concept of restricting food intake for weight loss has continued into the present day with various diet fads, such as intermittent fasting.

After the age of 40, the body's metabolism begins to slow down. This is why many older individuals struggle with weight loss. However, intermittent fasting can be an effective method for combating these side effects and promoting weight loss.

Intermittent fasting has not only been linked to rapid weight loss, but also to numerous health benefits, including improved blood sugar control, reduced inflammation, and enhanced brain health. If you are over 40, especially if you are a woman, you should also be aware of the effects of menopause on weight loss.

However, with intermittent fasting it is still possible to lose weight and improve overall health.

Menopause is an inevitable and natural part of the ageing process for women. It is the point in a woman's life when her menstrual cycle ceases and she can no longer conceive. Many women experience symptoms such as hot flashes and mood swings during this time.

In addition, weight gain is common during menopause because hormonal changes can lead to an increase in fat storage and a slowed metabolism.

But don't let this deter you from losing weight and enhancing your health! Intermittent fasting can still promote weight loss during menopause by controlling blood sugar and reducing inflammation.

After age 40, men also experience weight gain. This is frequently the result of a slowing metabolism, changes in hormone levels, and a decline in physical activity.

Men, like women, can combat these effects by adopting an intermittent fasting lifestyle. This will help maintain a healthy weight, control blood sugar levels, and reduce inflammation.

Chapter 7: What Benefits Does Fasting Offer?

Fasting has many benefits, including rapid weight loss, fat burning, and improved health. Intermittent fasting reduces insulin resistance, reduces inflammation, and improves heart health, according to studies. In addition, it has been shown to increase levels of human growth hormone, which can aid in muscle gain and fat loss.

Fasting can also improve mental clarity and concentration. In one study, intermittent fasting was shown to improve memory and brain function in mice, while in another, it may improve mood and reduce depressive symptoms.

It is a common misconception that fasting will cause you to lose muscle mass. When the body uses stored energy (fat) as fuel, it does not distinguish between muscle and fat. Consequently, it is essential to consume sufficient protein during mealtimes in order to preserve muscle mass. However, the body will not begin breaking down muscle for fuel until all of its stored energy has been consumed (fat).

Chapter 8: The Journey Of Intermittent Fasting – The Most Effective Method

Some people can immediately begin intermittent fasting with the flip of a switch, while others must gradually alter their eating habits. You inhabit a planet that has been overfed. As it is ingrained in our psychology to consume a large breakfast and snack throughout the day, it may take some time to adjust to consuming less food. Maybe you'll start intermittent fasting on Mondays, Wednesdays, and Fridays, or just on the weekends. whichever method is most effective for you to begin.

An expert, Greaves, states that IF is not appropriate for women who don't get enough sleep, don't eat enough or regularly, have irregular or nonexistent periods, have thyroid problems, have a history of present or past disordered eating, are under a great deal of stress, or have blood sugar issues. If your doctor or nutritionist has given you permission, start slowly. According to Greaves, research suggests that overnight fasting for 12 to 14 hours may result in metabolic improvements. "It is crucial to understand that you do not need to fast for 16 to 18 hours to reap the benefits." She recommends beginning with the time-restricted strategy rather than the 5:2 method, which restricts calories two days per week and encourages patients to binge on the remaining days.

Determine the number of hours between the time you finish eating at night and the time you start eating the following day. Start by extending your fast by one hour, then two, and so on. There are no calorie restrictions with time-restricted intermittent fasting. It is recommended to consume three well-balanced meals per day, with protein, carbohydrates with a high fibre content, and healthy fats. Those who have never been big breakfast eaters may find it easy to wait until 10 or 11 a.m. to eat, whereas others may awaken ravenous. It is essential to pay attention to the body and eat when it signals hunger. Intermittent fasting may be difficult for women who regularly exercise. If it's that time of the month and you're hungry, it will be difficult to fast. Can coffee assist in breaking the fast? Yes, technically, if it contains something. No calories are present in black coffee. But consider your goals: Are you trying to lose weight? If so, keep in mind that IF does not cause more weight loss than a calorie deficit, so a small amount of creamer in your coffee is likely safe. Are you doing this to control your blood sugar? In this case, a caramel latte is not the best way to start the day. The general course of action would be as follows:

Step 1: Eliminate breakfast

Breakfast is the most important meal of the day. Eliminating breakfast from your daily routine is the simplest and most effective way to begin intermittent fasting. The morning is when your body performs its own miracle. Food is the only interruption. The hormones cortisol and adrenaline rise in the morning to help you wake up, become alert, and produce energy.

Determine the optimal time to exercise in Step 2.

Contrary to popular belief, individuals can engage in physical activity while fasting. The best time of day for vigorous exercise is in the morning! You are young, healthy, and have hormonal equilibrium on your side. Afternoon and evening workouts aren't always as effective as they could be because you're exhausted from the day, preoccupied with whatever new work pressures have arisen, and resisting the urge to kick off your shoes and relax.

Step 3: Unwind. Your coffee (unsweetened) is still safe to consume.
Yes! Fortunately for coffee lovers around the world, their beloved morning ritual does not raise blood sugar or break a fast. If you cannot stomach the idea of drinking black coffee, add creamer... However, not excessively! Remember that your body must first metabolise the fat in creamer before returning to metabolising stored fat. What about coffee drinkers who require an artificial sweetener to mask bitterness? Zane, an expert on intermittent fasting, recommends avoiding all-natural

sweeteners such as honey, cane sugar, and agave nectar. Although they are "natural" carbohydrates, they rapidly increase blood sugar and insulin levels. Consequently, your body will no longer be in a state of fasting. If you desire a bit of sweetness in your coffee, use only a small amount of Stevia. The vast majority of artificial sugars are harmful because they stimulate cravings and trick the digestive system into expecting sugar that never arrives. This disrupts the fat-burning mechanism that fasting is meant to promote. Ultimately, the issue of coffee boils down to your goals. If you are attempting to lose fifty pounds, adding cream to your daily coffee may hinder your progress. In contrast, a sugary cup of coffee is far superior to a slice of cheesecake! It's all about finding the proper equilibrium.

This Fourth Step Is Also For Diabetics!

Every day, Zane (an expert on IF) interacts with diabetic clients who believe intermittent fasting is too dangerous. "I cannot think of a better way to control diabetes or treat its symptoms than figuring out how to introduce fasting," he says. Type two diabetes is a blood sugar imbalance disease, and intermittent fasting is an effective method for lowering and balancing blood sugar levels through healthier eating habits. The most effective method for enhancing glycemic control is fasting. Diabetics can use fasting to eliminate their need for medication and lessen the effects of diabetes if they take a planned, doctor-supervised approach.

Chapter 9: What If I Am Not Receiving Any Results?

What if, despite strictly adhering to the prescribed fasting regimen and doing nothing to increase insulin levels during the fasting period, you do not lose weight or inches? It's extremely discouraging to feel as though you're following all the rules but getting nowhere. If you are not losing weight, your body is doing everything it can to prevent it. First, consider the length of time you've been overweight. If you've struggled with this for a very long time, you may be very resistant to insulin. This could result in elevated insulin levels ALL DAY LONG, even when fasting as required. There are several possible outcomes if this applies to you. My first piece of advice is to give the benefits of fasting additional time to manifest. Restoring previous years' damage could take some time. Although it may appear that you are not making any progress, your body may be performing remarkable healing. Consider whether you had been steadily reducing your caloric intake prior to beginning your fasting schedule. If this is the case, your prolonged calorie restriction may have slowed your metabolism. Because your body attempts to protect you from starvation, a low-calorie diet should result in a slowed metabolism. You require fewer and fewer calories to maintain your weight over time. If you believe that this may be the case, allow some time for the metabolic-boosting benefits of fasting to take effect. Ensure that you are not restricting your eating throughout the entire eating window. The fasting period should speed up your metabolism, allowing you to lose weight once your body realises it is no longer starving.

It may be time to reconsider your diet if you have given it some time and still haven't noticed any changes. I am aware that I stated intermittent fasting allows you to eat whatever you want and is generally effective, but we are all unique. Even though 95% of people can eat whatever they want while intermittently fasting and losing weight, you could be one of the 5% of individuals who must alter their diet. In addition, I invented the 95%/5% statistic. Oops. I am unaware of anyone who has already submitted that information. That would make a fascinating research project.

If you have tried—and I mean really tried—to follow intermittent fasting and you are certain that you are fasting correctly but are not losing weight or inches, my first piece of advice would be to eliminate highly processed foods for a while and see if this makes a difference. As I mentioned in the chapter on what to eat, The Science of Skinny does an excellent job of explaining how to avoid processed foods and why you may want to consider doing so. Hopefully, this is the only modification you will have to make. Again, give yourself time to determine if it is effective.

If, after sufficient time, you do not experience any benefits, you may want to consider a low-carb, high-fat (LCHF) diet for a while. Those with type 2 diabetes or significant insulin resistance may need to take this step. Dr. Fung frequently discusses the LCHF lifestyle on his blog Intensive Dietary Management and in his book The Obesity Code. Combining the LCHF diet with intermittent fasting, he has achieved remarkable outcomes with his patients.

Adopting LCHF may, over time, help you reduce your high insulin levels and utilise fat storage (if this is, in fact, what is preventing you from losing weight) (if that is, indeed, what is keeping you from losing weight.) According to what I've read, combining LCHF with intermittent fasting should finally result in weight loss. Moreover, if the underlying insulin resistance has been resolved, you may be able to gradually reintroduce carbohydrates into your diet. You are aware of my fondness for carbohydrates and my inability to imagine life without them; therefore, I do not make this recommendation lightly. My personal position is "delay, don't deny," and I would never advise anyone to restrict their food intake. Although it appears that some individuals require this additional step, I would not be doing you a favour by not bringing it up.

Another strategy for addressing underlying insulin resistance is prolonged fasting. Dr. Fung and Jimmy Moore discuss longer fasts in their collaborative book The Complete Guide to Fasting. This book focuses primarily on LCHF, but it also discusses how to adopt longer fasts and why you would want to do so. If you are interested in learning more, I recommend reading their book. When longer fasts are undertaken, a physician with knowledge of fasting techniques should be present. Stress and other variables, such as medications, may also affect weight loss. Medications that have a reputation for causing weight gain will likely make weight loss more difficult. Never stop taking a medication without first consulting your doctor. Due to the effects of excessive cortisol, your body may resist weight loss if you are under a great deal of stress. As noted in the insulin chapter, our bodies rely heavily on hormones, which regulate a variety of underappreciated processes. Make an effort to reduce your stress levels and examine your sleep hygiene. It's easier to say than to do, right? Most importantly, you must establish that you ARE NOT receiving results if you believe you are not. In my experience, people who claim they are not seeing results have either not given themselves enough time or have unrealistic expectations. As I've indicated, intermittent fasting is not a rapid weight loss method. The fact that weight loss is not occurring quickly does not indicate that your body is not responding appropriately. Toss the scale or keep in mind the importance of weighing oneself daily and then averaging the weekly results for comparison purposes. In addition to aiding in weight loss, intermittent fasting has a plethora of additional benefits, even if you don't notice them immediately.

Chapter 10: Positive Aspects Of The Omad Diet

OMAD can be an effective strategy for rapid and permanent weight loss. The majority of individuals find that it suppresses their appetite sufficiently to make consuming fewer calories practically effortless.

There is also a hormonal component to the weight loss potential of OMAD.

Daily fasting for 23 hours reduces storage hormones such as insulin (which converts blood sugar into fat), making it easy to switch into fat-burning mode.

Your body will burn fat for 23 hours per day while gaining one hour of muscle.

The majority of people find that this diet is quite effective for maintaining muscle mass while losing weight.

According to one study, intermittent fasting preserved muscle mass better than a "normal" diet of equal calories.

In turn, muscle can aid in weight loss because most muscles burn fat while at rest.

In comparison, the traditional American diet does an excellent job of increasing blood sugar and preventing the use of fat as a fuel source.

It is not surprising that the majority of SAD adherents are thin or, at best, obese.

Your metabolic rate may increase during fasting.

Contrary to popular belief, fasting appears to increase metabolism rather than decrease it. According to multiple studies, fasting can increase the metabolism by 3.6% to 14%.

OMAD also stimulates the production of ketones within the body. These energy molecules, including beta-hydroxybutyrate, are derived from fat and offer numerous health benefits. Ketones are especially advantageous for the brain, where they help regulate neurotransmission and other aspects of cognitive health.

OMAD Diet Benefit No. 2: It Reduces Inflammation

Chronic inflammation has been linked to virtually all diseases. According to experts, it is responsible for the majority of today's chronic diseases.

Thankfully, fasting can immediately reduce inflammation.

The mechanism is straightforward: during a fast, the body is not preoccupied with digestion and nutrient absorption, allowing it to focus on reducing inflammatory markers.

Even the intestinal lining can benefit from rest; it spends a great deal of time repairing, which further reduces inflammation.

Ketones fuel your mitochondria and stimulate the production of new mitochondria; therefore, entering a ketogenic state can help reduce inflammation.

Mitophagy is a mechanism that is anti-inflammatory and anti-aging.

OMAD's ability to reduce inflammation is likely the reason why it appears to increase longevity. According to Roden's research, eating less frequently can increase longevity by as much as 80 percent.

OMAD Diet Advantage #3: Better Mental Health
Extensive fasting has been shown in studies to stimulate the production of neurohormones that improve mental health directly.

One such hormone activated by fasting is Brain-Derived Neurotrophic Factor

(BDNF), which is extremely neuroplastic.

Increased levels of BDNF have been linked to improved mood, cognition, and creativity.

Many individuals claim that OMAD keeps them alert throughout the day, adding a mental benefit.

If your 'healthy' lunch makes you lethargic and unmotivated, the OMAD diet offers a straightforward solution: skip it!

Fourth OMAD Diet Benefit: A Younger Appearance

OMAD is renowned for its ability to reverse the biological clock. Many individuals report that their skin becomes plumper and more radiant after daily fasting. And new research suggests that this is not merely a placebo effect caused by hunger.

A recent study found that a 24-hour fast increased anti-aging chemicals such as human growth hormone (HGH) by 1,300 to 2,000%.

This unique hormone is necessary for the development of muscle fibres, connective tissue, and skin. It is most likely responsible for the smoother wrinkles and brighter complexion that many OMAD users observe in the mirror.

Dietary Freedom is OMAD Diet Benefit #5!

This final advantage is more pragmatic. OMAD provides significant nutritional and logistical flexibility to individuals with demanding schedules.

No more waking up early to prepare breakfast; no more settling for subpar lunches at the office; no more contemplating eating on the go with the OMAD diet.

Simply consume one large, well-balanced meal per day, wherever and whenever you please.

Many people find OMAD mentally liberating because they are not preoccupied with food during the day.

However, this only works if sufficient calories are consumed from healthy, whole foods. At McDonald's, ordering half the menu will not suffice.

Chapter 11: How Is Intermittent Fasting Effective?

Intermittent fasting (IF) is a method of eating that alternates periods of fasting with predetermined food windows. When compared to traditional "diets," IF places less emphasis on what or how much you eat and more emphasis on when you eat. The meal's quality is important, but it is not the primary concern.

To fast is to abstain from all caloric intake. Due to the lack of calories, water, herbal tea, and black coffee are acceptable beverages (or they contain trace amounts). However, anything with calories is prohibited. Fasting is not new, but intermittent fasting appears to be a hot topic in all health circles. It has always been an indispensable aspect of spirituality and religion. Fasting has been a health trend for quite some time, although it has only recently gained widespread popularity.

Its adaptability to your lifestyle is one reason for its widespread popularity. There is not just one correct way to practise intermittent fasting; there are a variety of methods (which you can learn about below). Compared to a typical calorie-restricted diet, it may appear less restrictive. Fasting is beneficial because it aligns with our natural physiology, according to specialists in intermittent fasting. However, this is still debatable IF proponents contend that humans were designed to endure long periods without food.

In any case, intermittent fasting may help you reduce your calorie intake by permitting you to go longer without eating, especially overnight (especially if you are prone to late-night snacking). As you will discover, however, there are additional benefits of fasting besides weight loss.

How does intermittent fasting affect women's health?

Despite its widespread use, we must acknowledge that the majority of IF research participants are male. Few studies take the biology of women into account (as is the case for a lot of medical research, unfortunately). Moreover, given that women's and men's physiologies are quite different, it makes sense that intermittent fasting would affect us differently.

In one of the few studies with both male and female participants, it was discovered that while IF improved blood sugar responses in men, it worsened them in women.

This implies that women should never attempt too quickly, correct? No, but some individuals, particularly those who frequently fast, should not. There are methods of fasting that are suitable for women's biology, for those who can safely practise intermittent fasting.

Consider the overall benefits and drawbacks of intermittent fasting for women.

Chapter 12: The benefits of intermittent fasting include:

The benefits of intermittent fasting are derived not only from eating less, but also from metabolic changes that occur when you go longer without food.

Autophagy is the primary adaptation induced by fasting. When nutrients are scarce, your body's self-cleaning system, known as autophagy, activates. In order to preserve cellular and metabolic health, healthy cells replace unhealthy ones as old or damaged ones are eliminated.

Autophagy is associated with longevity and the prevention of chronic diseases. Fasting may be an effective natural method for boosting autophagy activity, which declines with age.

Autophagy is one of the benefits of intermittent fasting, but there are numerous other fascinating research findings, such as:

Numerous studies have shown the benefits of intermittent fasting. In addition to limiting late-night mindless eating, research suggests that people who practise intermittent fasting lose weight just as effectively as those who restrict their caloric intake without feeling deprived.

accelerated fat loss If you reduce your carbohydrate intake, your body uses alternative fuel sources. After depleting your meagre carbohydrate reserves, you can use fat as a substitute. According to a number of studies, fasting activates the metabolic switch that enables fat to be used as fuel, thereby increasing fat burning.

Mental well-being. Particularly in relation to ageing, fasting may enhance cognitive function. Even though it has been studied primarily in animal models, it may also aid in slowing neurodegeneration, the progressive loss of brain cells.

Longevity. Autophagy can reduce oxidative damage and promote healthy ageing by promoting cellular health through the elimination of old, damaged cells.

Heart health. A healthy cholesterol level affects your risk of heart disease, and fasting may help you maintain it.

Insulin resistance and insulin resistance. Both calorie restriction and fasting may improve body weight, insulin levels, and insulin resistance.

Immunity. The process of autophagy, which occurs during fasting, may have a positive effect on the production of healthy white blood cells.

Inflammation. Numerous studies have demonstrated that fasting reduces markers of oxidative and inflammatory stress.

Chapter 13: Consequences and hazards of intermittent fasting

With all of these potential benefits, incorporating fasting into your daily routine seems like a no-brainer; in fact, this is the appeal that has so many people participating. There are a few things to consider before beginning, especially for women.

Before beginning any type of fast, you should consult a healthcare professional, as you would with any other significant dietary change. Even a mild fast can be dangerous, especially for those with a history of an eating disorder or disordered eating pattern.

You may have diabetes or hypoglycemia, especially if you use blood sugar-lowering medications.

Having trouble gaining sufficient weight or overcoming nutritional deficiencies.

electrolyte abnormalities in the past, especially during longer fasts.

Even though you may still be able to fast if you belong to one of these groups, it is more important to get the proper guidance to determine whether it is safe for you. If you have a history of disordered eating or an eating disorder, it is highly recommended that you consult with a trained health professional prior to beginning. The benefits may outweigh the potential risks.

Chapter 14: What Intermittent Fasting Entails

Intermittent fasting is a period of food abstinence for a number of hours, including the night, from all caloric foods and beverages. However, it is recommended to consume up to 3 litres of water, coffee, or tea without sugar or milk. The optimal frequency is one fast per week, such as beginning on Monday night and concluding on Tuesday evening. The plan is to consume two light meals during this time period. But where does this insane notion originate? And the reverse inquiry should be: why do I eat at regular hours and three to five times per day?

Our ancestors, the hunter-gatherers, endured fasting periods without experiencing famine because the slow periods coincided with the time needed to find food. You eat when you are hungry, like wild animals, and not according to an education or ideas implanted by industrialists to consume you. On the other hand, your body is designed to support unprocessed foods provided by Mother Nature. As a result of evolution and industrialization, however, you are forced to digest a wide variety of foods. Fasting makes it possible to clean up a small portion of this entire website.

Chapter 15: How Intermittent Fasting Works Physiologically

In a world where cardiovascular disease, hypertension, and diabetes have become masters, achieving and maintaining a healthy weight is important, if not crucial. However, achieving this healthy weight is not always simple. For some, losing weight can be a very difficult task. There are times when the most extreme methods, including strict diets, caloric restriction, and physical activity, are employed. However, they can be ineffective in terms of long-term weight loss. Thankfully, intermittent fasting remains a little-known but effective treatment option.

The fundamentals of intermittent fasting

Intermittent fasting is a variation on traditional fasting, which involves starvation. It differs from other diets in that it alternates periods of fasting with normal eating. The implementation of this trick does not require a change in diet or consideration of a low-calorie diet. It will only be necessary to eat at predetermined times and to fast between meals while consuming adequate amounts of water. It is not technically a diet, but rather a food behaviour.

• INTERMITTENT FASTING RECIPES

Aside from the period of Lent, you may consume whatever and as much food as you please. That sounds seductive at first, obviously. However, you should make wise food choices. Fast food or unhealthy ready meals should only be served in the most dire of circumstances. By selecting low-carbohydrate recipes with high satiety levels, the RIGHT diet can increase the success of interval harvesting. And that is precisely how I intend to assist you.

• HOW DOES INTERMITTENT FASTING WORK

16:8 intermittent fasting and 5:2 intermittent fasting are the two most common types. The first form fasts for sixteen hours per day. Then you can eat within an 8-hour window. However, one should keep in mind that, obviously, eating does not equate to fasting. If at all possible, restrict the number of meals to two or three. In contrast, during the 5:2-Intermittent fast, you eat normally five days per week and fast two days per week. On the two days of fasting, women consume no more than 500 calories per day, while men consume no more than 600 calories per day.

Each person must determine which form of intermittent fasting is optimal for them. Professionals frequently find the 5:2 formula to be a good fit because it allows them to eat normally five days per week. In addition, the two days of fasting make up for nutritional mistakes and lavish business lunches. In my personal experience, it can be difficult to go without food for an entire day. Therefore, I recommend the 16:8 form, particularly for beginners.

- Why is intermittent fasting so powerful?

The human body is not designed to consume food continuously. It is overwhelmed by the constant availability of food in the modern era. In the past, it was common practise to have a nutritious breakfast in the morning and not eat again until bedtime. In between, there was at most something to drink or a little something like a piece of fruit. Because the body was no longer constantly engaged with food intake and digestion, it was able to focus on other tasks, such as cell regeneration. This decreased the risk of chronic diseases that have become prevalent in the modern era. Intermittent fasting is based on this age-old principle of food consumption: you eat only during certain time windows and fast at other times.

Chapter 16: What Happens When We Fast Your Body Always Needs Energy.

Even when you are resting or sleeping, your body is working to maintain the health of your heart, lungs, and all other vital systems. Nevertheless, we assert that fasting — when you do not provide your body with a new source of energy — is advantageous. Fasting is recommended for weight management, cellular repair, inflammation reduction, cognitive enhancement, and disease prevention and mitigation.

Examining the five stages of fasting within the body will help us determine why this is the case.

Experts, such as physicians and nutritionists, spend years deciphering the complexities of this story. I lack the required knowledge. My life experiences have convinced me that intermittent fasting is beneficial. What follows is a compilation of what I've learned over the years from experts.

After a meal, the fed state lasts for four hours. When you are in the fed state, your body is primarily concerned with digesting and absorbing nutrients from the food you have consumed.

You are consuming energy in the form of food, which is being digested into the necessary proteins, fats, and carbohydrates for your body.

For the body to absorb these essential nutrients, they must be further broken down. Proteins are broken down into amino acids, which contribute to body function and muscle growth. Fats are converted into fatty acids, which are then utilised in the synthesis of hormones and cell membranes. Carbohydrates are converted into glucose (blood sugar), which is your cells' primary source of energy.

In the fed state, blood glucose levels increase.

The body stores nutrients it does not immediately require in preparation for times of scarcity. The accumulation of fatty acids within fat cells. Unutilized amino acids are capable of being converted to fat for storage. As glycogen, glucose is stored in the liver and fat cells. In addition to aiding in digestion, the pancreas secretes insulin when food is consumed. Insulin is a hormone that aids in the transport of glucose into cells. As you likely know, diabetes is a disease that impairs insulin's function.

Because the fed state is triggered whenever food is consumed, it is essential to consume only water or non-caloric beverages during a fast.

Overeating is also a problem for people with diabetes or pre-diabetes because it causes the body to produce excessive amounts of insulin.

When you stop eating, however, your body enters a state known as early fasting after four hours. This has also been referred to as the catabolic state, which is fine, but what does it mean?

Catabolic state is related to metabolism. The process by which your body uses energy, or metabolism, has two states: anabolic and catabolic. The anabolic state occurs when the body's processes are focused on growth. The Fed is an anabolic state.

The catabolic state is characterised by the breakdown of nutrients to fuel other bodily functions. During the catabolic state, your cells' glycogen (stored glucose) will be utilised for energy first. The body then begins to burn stored energy as fat.

As the body begins to burn glycogen energy from fat, you may need to urinate more frequently. This is due to the fact that each gramme of glycogen contains three grammes of water.

Similarly, when you urinate, you excrete electrolytes, which are minerals that conduct electrical signals throughout the body to enable nerve and muscle function and to help maintain the balance of bodily fluids. This is why it is essential to consume a lot of water when fasting.

When your body begins to derive the majority of its energy from fat cells rather than glucose, you have entered a state known as ketosis. When ketosis occurs depends on the types of foods consumed.

Some individuals will enter ketosis near the end of the early fasting state. Ketosis will occur sooner if you consume more fat and protein and less starch and carbohydrates.

Achieving ketosis is one of the objectives of fasting.

In ketosis, the body produces molecules known as ketones or ketone bodies. These ketones are derived from fatty acids and serve as an alternative fuel source to glucose. Ketones produce more energy with fewer inflammatory byproducts than glucose, which contributes to greater mental clarity and reduced symptoms of conditions such as diabetes and cardiovascular disease.

Throughout the 12:12 and 16:8 forms of intermittent fasting, you will experience the early fasting state.

If you are already in ketosis, the process will now speed up. If you are not following a moderate, low-carbohydrate diet while intermittent fasting, you may not enter ketosis for 16–24 hours. When you enter the fasting state, you will experience ketosis regardless of your diet.

During ketosis, you will begin to feel less hungry, which will make it easier to adhere to a fasting programme.

When you are in ketosis, exercise is also recommended. During ketosis, it is possible to increase the concentration of ketone in the blood from 0.05–0.1 millimoles to 5–7 millimoles. Aerobic exercise, such as running, will significantly accelerate the process.

Additionally, if you fast for 24 hours, your glycogen stores will be depleted. In addition to burning fat, your body will also speed up the autophagy process, which is desirable.

When certain bodily processes are activated, others are deactivated or minimised. When food is readily available and you are eating, one of the things that occurs is that the body reduces autophagy.

The term autophagy is derived from the Greek words auto (self) and phagein (to eat). Autophagy is the process by which cells clean themselves by consuming themselves, breaking down and reusing old, damaged, and abnormal components.

Autophagy has multiple health benefits.

You may have heard that every seven years the body regenerates itself. This is due to a process known as apoptosis. As your body's cells age, they naturally die and are replaced by new ones. Autophagy is a transitional process. Damaged or abnormal cells that are too young to die are repaired.

Autophagy degrades damaged or abnormal cellular components, repairing them and releasing reusable constituents, such as amino acids, fatty acids, and glucose.

Furthermore, autophagy has an anti-inflammatory effect.

Surely you are familiar with inflammation caused by minor cuts. It occurs both inside and outside the body when the immune system is activated in response to an injury.

Some diseases overstimulate the immune system, resulting in persistent inflammation. This is a problem for individuals with rheumatoid arthritis, Type 2 diabetes, cancer, Alzheimer's disease, cardiovascular disease, and even asthma. Autophagy's anti-inflammatory effect can provide relief. There is even speculation that it can help prevent or treat cancer.

Due to the fact that autophagy is stimulated during the fasting state, increased autophagy results in healthier cells.

This explains how intermittent fasting can extend your lifespan. Since 1945, studies on mice have demonstrated this effect on longevity, and now studies on humans demonstrate the same effect.

A 2006 study of residents living in senior housing, conducted over a three-year period, compared a control group who consumed the daily recommended amount of calories to a test group who fasted every other day. On the day of fasting, they only consumed 56% of the recommended daily calories. The following day, they ate 144% of their daily caloric intake. Both groups consumed the same amount of food over the course of the two days, but only one group fasted.

Chapter 17: Diet & Nutrition

As you likely already know, nutrition is a crucial component of any health and fitness journey. The problem is that we know what to eat most of the time! You are likely aware that vegetables are healthy, that meat contains protein, and that processed foods are generally unhealthy. I will not reiterate the adage to avoid bread and pasta, which you have heard a hundred times. However, we will discuss two essential electrolytes that many people are deficient in, as well as how much fat, protein, and carbohydrates you should consume for optimal results.

Focus initially on becoming accustomed to your window. You will obtain rapid results. As soon as you are accustomed to the 16:8 way of life, continue to develop new ideas for different outcomes.

Protein, Carbs, and Fats

As stated previously, the objective of the game is to deplete glycogen stores, forcing the body to utilise fat. The objective is to gradually acclimatise the body to using fat as its primary source of fuel so that it can remain lean throughout the year. This is best achieved by consuming more fat and fewer carbohydrates. Protein must be consumed in moderation because excessive protein can be converted into glucose and stored as glycogen. Some common macros are displayed below. I would like to emphasise that IF can be utilised by anyone, regardless of whether they are ketogenic or not.

Always consult your physician before making dietary changes.

Starter: Avoid processed sugars.

Instead of macronutrients, a beginner should incorporate resistant starches and eliminate refined sugars.

Resistant starches

Resistant starches cannot be metabolised like soluble fibres. They aid in lowering blood sugar levels and insulin resistance, among other things. These alternatives to conventional sources of carbohydrates are superior.

Examples:

Sweet potato and yams are substituted for potatoes. Oatmeal rather than cereal Substitute cooked and cooled rice for warm rice. Bananas in the vicinity of other fruits

Keep in mind that if a substance remains solid at room temperature, it almost certainly contains saturated fat. Even fats that are liquid at room temperature become hydrogenated when heated.

Dairy and Animal Products

If you are not allergic to animals or a vegetarian, animal products are an excellent way to meet your protein and fat needs. However, before consuming them, keep a few things in mind.

Cattle, for instance, did not evolve to consume grains, so they are given medications to prevent them from experiencing the negative effects on their bodies. This practise is inhumane and harmful to your health, and companies engage in it to save money.

Dr. Gundry has written the book, The Plant Paradox. It's a wonderful read!

Guidelines for Fruit

There is so much contradictory information about fruit that this book should address it specifically.

Fruit contains an abundance of sugar.

On a molecular level, your cells do not divide foods like chocolate and fruit into "healthy" and "unhealthy" categories. Quite simply, glucose is glucose. Any other sugar, including fructose, dextrose, and any other word beginning with "ose," is converted to glucose and utilised in the same manner.

If you want to lose weight, you should only consume fruit in small quantities and only when it is in season. During the winter months when food is scarce, fruit is a bulking agent for our bodies. Our bodies are oblivious to the fact that we live in a society where food is readily available year-round. If you regularly consume fruit, you're signalling to your body that winter is approaching and that it should begin storing food. Here's how to lose weight with fruit:

Avoid eating fruit smoothies.

• Consume fruit immediately after exercise with a protein shake. •

94

Consume fruit without a protein source at all times.

Fruit smoothies are loaded with sugar. Because of the sugar content, the beverage has no antioxidant properties. Smoothies made with leafy greens offer the same benefits. Eating fruit with it is a great way to increase insulin levels after exercise so that muscle cells can absorb the protein shake. I know that spikes in insulin are usually bad news when fasting to lose weight, but in this case, they will make lean muscle gain worse because insulin also helps cells absorb protein. Make sure to pair fruit with a protein source like nuts if you plan to eat it as a snack. You'll get longer-lasting energy and prevent energy loss later in the day because this will slow the sugars' absorption into the bloodstream.

Guidelines for Breakfast

Breakfast is another contentious subject that merits special attention. It's common knowledge that breakfast is the day's most important meal. Although true, you don't have to eat breakfast every morning.

Breaking your fast is what the word "breakfast" means. Break quickly.

Think of breakfast as your first meal from now on, no matter what time you eat it. For instance, I eat breakfast between 1 and 2 p.m.

Traditionally, people have found that starting their 16:8 eating window later in the day makes it more accessible. Choose the window that best suits your needs—this is not gospel. So, don't worry if you don't like breakfast because you can still lose weight.

The most important thing I can tell you about your first meal is to ensure it has a lot of protein and fat but little carbs.

This is because what you eat first will determine how much fuel your body burns throughout the day. You will experience unpleasant sugar cravings, energy dips, and brain fog from a carbohydrate breakfast that primes the body to seek sugary sources. You'll feel fuller for extended periods if you eat a breakfast high in protein and fats. It has also been demonstrated that eating this kind of breakfast at the beginning of the day increases serotonin levels, which in turn helps with depression and anxiety.

So....

Avoid resistant starches in this meal as well.

Summary

Use the formula listed under protein guidelines to calculate your daily protein needs accurately. Resistant starches are better for blood sugar levels and promote insulin sensitivity. Cooking with saturated fat is healthier than using hydrogenated oils like vegetable oil. It is saturated fat if it stays solid at average room temperature. To give you the ideal beginning without overpowering you, I will discuss two significant electrolytes you can add to your eating regimen TODAY.

Potassium Muscle Cramps and Tightness
When we experience muscle cramps, we frequently hear that we lack magnesium or water. This is true, but a lack of potassium may contribute to muscle tightness. This is because we require significantly more potassium than magnesium daily.

Among the symptoms of low potassium are:

Tightness in the muscles Swollen ankles Cravings for sugar (yes, low potassium can cause cravings for sugar) (yes, low potassium can cause cravings for sugar) Beet tops, avocado, spinach, lime beans, potato, and brussels sprouts are good sources of potassium. Try including some of these foods more frequently to get more potassium. Potatoes and lima beans should be avoided due to their high carbohydrate content. It is best to consume these in moderation.

Chapter 18: Lose Weight By Modifying Your Cooking

Here are some suggestions to help you lose your first 10 pounds through simple dietary changes. Similarly, the manner in which food is prepared affects its nutritional value.

TIP No. 1: Boil vegetables as opposed to roasting or frying them. Probably the best way to consume vegetables such as carrots, broccoli, cauliflower, and cabbage is by steaming them.

Instead of frying these foods in lard or oil, consider baking them. When food is baked, it is not cooked in the same amount of fat and oil as when it is fried.

In Tip 3, replace the oil with nonstick cooking spray. Moreover, nonstick pans require minimal to no oil.

TIP #4: Avoid meals with no or minimal fat content. Despite their widespread availability, many foods are not particularly nutritious. Many of these meals are sweetened with chemicals or carbohydrates to improve their flavour. Even if the body converts these chemicals and carbohydrates into sugar, they still result in the production of fat.

5. Refrain from succumbing to crash diets Your health will suffer as a result, and in the end, they will cause more harm than good. In most cases, you will lose a few pounds temporarily, but as soon as you stop, the weight will return and even increase. You eventually reach a point where you are unable to survive on such a diet and must abandon it.

Chew liquid meals, sweets, and ice cream eight to twelve times prior to swallowing. The addition of saliva to the food aids in the digestion of sugar. Simply swallowing food without chewing completely fills the stomach with undigested food that lacks the necessary health benefits.

The seventh tip suggests using premium extra virgin olive oil for cooking. Although it is more expensive than vegetable oil, the higher health benefits justify the higher cost. Olive oil strengthens arterial walls, thereby decreasing the risk of heart attack and stroke. Furthermore, it has been associated with a reduced risk of coronary heart disease.

Chapter 19: Exercises For Fat Loss

Two things you must do in order to lose weight are eating healthy foods and drinking enough pure water, and one of them has already been discussed in detail. The second thing you must do is to get your body moving. You can exercise without purchasing a gym membership. There are, in fact, a number of daily activities and exercises you can perform on your own to help your body begin losing weight.

TIP #1: Weigh yourself prior to beginning exercise, but don't use the numbers to gauge your weight loss progress. The weight you carry fluctuates throughout the day. If you weigh yourself every day, you may decide to quit.

The most reliable indicator that you're losing weight is how well your clothes fit.

When you begin to float around in your clothes, you'll know that eating well and exercising are helping you. Another sign that you're losing weight is that the location where your belt usually fastens is shifting; this is a positive sign.

Reward yourself if you consistently monitor your weight and clothing size. Purchase a new pair of running shoes or jeans for yourself.

This can help you maintain motivation as you pursue your weight loss objectives.

TIP #4: Take a day off from exercise to allow your body to heal and recover. Each week, your body requires a day of rest.

TIP #5: You can maintain your weight with three 30-minute workouts per week, but you need at least four 30-minute workouts per week before you can begin to lose weight; five workouts per week is preferable.

Learn about workout routines and simple home projects. There is a wealth of information available about exercise, and you can choose what will help you achieve your weight loss objectives most effectively. Consult the Internet or books on health and fitness that are available at your local library or bookstore for additional information on how to burn the desired number of calories per week.

Find a workout companion who shares your commitment to fitness and weight loss. Having someone to feel responsible to is an advantage of finding a committed partner. Knowing that someone is waiting for you makes it easier to rise and exercise. Why would you want to make your workout partner stand up?

TIP #8: Take a break when your body signals that it has had enough. Following some physical activity, you will begin to perceive signals from your body. This is especially important when beginning a workout regimen.

If you choose to extend your workouts, do so gradually. Your workout intensity remains unchanged.

Choose an exercise regimen that complements your lifestyle.

Everyone has a distinct lifestyle and pursues a variety of occupations. There is no fixed duration during which you must exercise. If you find that exercising right before bedtime calms you, you should do so. It's also great if you enjoy working out in the morning because it helps you wake up. Some individuals enjoy exercising during their lunch break because it is the only time available to them or because their jobs are stressful.

Instead of standing still, you should move around. If you can move, you should do so. Pacers benefit greatly from frequent movement because it keeps them healthy. Pacing improves mental clarity.